# LIGHTLY

## HOW TO LIVE A SIMPLE, SERENE AND STRESS FREE LIFE

**LINDEN DOYLE**

## INTRODUCTION

Stress is an ordinary response the body has when changes happen. It can react to these progressions physically, rationally, or inwardly.

As we all know, Stress can pose a major challenge to our health and well-being and as such has to be avoided and dealt with as it may lead to certain complications in the body system and it also leads to depression

This book serves as a guideline and teaches you how to deal, cope, manage and live with stress.

# TABLE OF CONTENTS

WHAT IS STRESS..................................................1

HOW DOES STRESS AFFECT THE WELL BEING............................................................2

SYMPTOMS OF STRESS .............................3

PHYSICAL SIDEFFECTS OF STRESS................4

CONSEQUENCES OF LONG TERM STRESS................................................................5

LIVING A STRESS FREE LIFE.........................6

DEALING WITH STRESS................................7

# CHAPTER ONE

## WHAT IS STRESS

Stress is an ordinary response the body has when changes happen. It can react to these progressions physically, rationally, or inwardly.

### What is stress?

Stress is the body's response to any change that requires a modification or reaction. The body responds to these progressions with physical, mental, and passionate reactions. Stress is a typical piece of life.

You can experience worry from your condition, your body, and your musings. Indeed, even positive life changes, for example, advancement, a home loan, or the introduction of a kid produce stress.

## CHAPTER TWO

## HOW DOES STRESS AFFECT THE WELL BEING

The human body is intended to experience stress and respond to it. Stress can be certain, keeping us alert, persuaded, and prepared to stay away from peril. Stress winds up adverse when an individual faces ceaseless difficulties without alleviation or unwinding between stressors. Therefore, the individual progresses toward becoming exhausted and stress-related strain manufactures. The body's autonomic sensory system has a worked in stress reaction that makes physiological changes enable the body to battle upsetting circumstances. This stress reaction, otherwise called the "battle or flight reaction", is initiated in the event of a crisis. In any case, this reaction can turn out to be incessantly actuated during delayed times of stress.

Drawn out initiation of the stress reaction causes mileage on the body – both physical and enthusiastic.

Stress that proceeds without alleviation can prompt a condition called trouble – a negative stress response.

Trouble can bother the body's inward equalization or harmony, prompting physical indications, for example, cerebral pains, an annoyed stomach, raised pulse, chest torment, sexual brokenness, and issues resting. Enthusiastic issues can likewise result from trouble.

These issues incorporate despondency, alarm assaults, or different types of tension and stress. Research recommends that stress additionally can expedite or compound certain indications or infections. Stress is connected to 6 of the main sources of death: coronary illness, malignancy, lung infirmities, mishaps, cirrhosis of the liver, and suicide.

Stress likewise winds up destructive when individuals participate in the urgent utilization of substances or practices to attempt to ease their stress. These substances or practices incorporate nourishment, liquor, tobacco, drugs, betting, sex, shopping, and the Internet. Instead of mitigating the stress and restoring the body to a casual express, these substances and urgent practices will in general keep the body in a focused on state and cause more issues.

The upset individual ends up caught in an endless loop.

## CHAPTER THREE

## SYMPTOMS OF STRESS

What Are the Symptoms of Stress?

Stress can be a challenge to most parts of your life, including your feelings, practices, thinking capacity, and physical wellbeing.

No piece of the body is invulnerable. Be that as it may, on the grounds that individuals handle pressure in an unexpected way, side effects of pressure can differ. Indications can be obscure and might be equivalent to those brought about by ailments. So it is essential to talk about them with your primary care physician. You may encounter any of the accompanying indications of stress.

**Emotional side effects of pressure include:**

- Ending up effectively upset, disappointed, and ill humored
- Feeling overpowered, similar to you are losing control or need to take control
- Experiencing issues unwinding and calming your brain
- Feeling awful about yourself (low confidence), forlorn, useless, and discouraged

- Maintaining a strategic distance from others

## CHAPTER FOUR

## PHYSICAL SIDEFFECTS OF STRESS

- Low vitality
- Cerebral pains
- Resentful stomach, including looseness of the bowels, obstruction, and sickness
- Throbs, torments, and tense muscles
- Chest torment and fast heartbeat
- A sleeping disorder
- Visit colds and contaminations
- Loss of sexual want or potentially capacity

- Anxiety and shaking, ringing in the ear, cold or sweat-soaked hands and feet
- Dry mouth and trouble gulping
- Grasped jaw and granulating teeth
- Intellectual side effects of pressure include:
- Consistent stressing
- Dashing contemplations
- Absent mindedness and disruption
- Failure to center
- Misguided thinking
- Being critical or seeing just the negative side

Behavioral indications of stress include:

- Changes in craving - either not eating or eating excessively
- Stalling and keeping away from obligations
- Expanded utilization of liquor, medications, or cigarettes
- Showing progressively anxious practices, for example, nail gnawing, squirming, and pacing

# CHAPTER FIVE

# CONSEQUENCES OF LONG TERM STRESS

A little pressure from time to time isn't something to be worried about. Continuous, constant pressure, nonetheless, can cause or intensify numerous genuine medical issues, including:

Psychological well-being issues, for example, wretchedness, tension, and character issue

Cardiovascular sickness, including coronary illness, hypertension, unusual heart rhythms, heart assaults, and stroke

Corpulence and other dietary problems

**Menstrual issues**

Sexual brokenness, for example, feebleness and untimely discharge in men and loss of sexual want in the two people

Skin and hair issues, for example, skin break out, psoriasis, and dermatitis, and changeless male pattern baldness

Gastrointestinal issues, for example, GERD, gastritis, ulcerative colitis, and bad tempered colon

# CHAPTER SIX

## LIVING A STRESS FREE LIFE

That is better, would it say it isn't? Presently, focus on the grounds that these all around kept privileged insights have been utilized by the experts for a considerable length of time to deal with their pressure. They are simple methods you can apply anyplace and might enable you to lessen your feeling of anxiety drastically when your uneasiness level ascents up.

Take a full breath and read on.

### 1. it's about viewpoint. No, truly, it is.

You've heard a gazillion times: the glass is either half unfilled or half full. You pick the manner in which you need to take a gander at life. More often than not, stress is made up by deceptions and negative self-talk.

See, if the things you are agonizing over right presently can't be fathomed in the following 2 hours or on the off chance that you have positively no power over the circumstance, for example, the climate or a deferred train, at that point let it go. Have sympathy for your circumstance as opposed to pounding yourself or accusing others. Move your point of view. Grasp whatever life tosses at you with appreciation. See the master plan and attempt to see what life is giving you rather than what is deficient. Go help another person, move your consideration off of yourself and offer it to another person. It's difficult to be pushed when life is significant.

**2. In the event that you can direct your breath, you can manage basically anything throughout everyday life.** The intensity of your breath is enormous. Your breath is the one component that associates you to the remainder of us, it keeps you alive and encourages you explore the physical and enthusiastic difficulties of life. Normally, when you're irate, pushed or frightened the mood of your breath quickens, now and then so much that you can barely explain a word.

In any case, here is the thing. You have every one of the assets accessible to you at each minute to hinder your breath and re-focus yourself. You should simply to concentrate to your heart focus, perhaps close your eyes and take even breathes in and breathes out until your pulse goes down. It's extremely simple and anyone can do it. It just expects you to concentrate all your consideration onto your breath for a couple of minutes. What's more, recollect, on the off chance that you have control over your breath, you are most likely substantially more dominant than you might suspect you are.

## 3. Respect your basic beliefs.

Uprightness, genuineness, mental fortitude, energy, generosity, regard and responsibility. You have a lot of guiding principle that you live by. These qualities, lead you through life, help you in your everyday basic leadership and shape your mentality towards others. Being aware of your guiding principle and tailing them is critical. Frequently, on the off chance that you or another person neglects to respect these qualities, a colossal measure of pressure and stress is made. You can feel regretful, lacking and embarrassed.

Respecting your qualities liberates your cognizant personality and add to hold your worry under tight restraints. Support yourself and remain steadfast, your wellbeing relies upon it!

## 4. Give yourself a hug

Possibly not truly, alright? In any case, feel free to clean up, light candles, consume incense, play your main tune on rehash, call a companion, book a back rub, go on a retreat. Do whatever you have to do to feel like you are dealt with. Being worried can make you feel ignored, depleted and defenseless.

Cutting time to back off and be available to yourself is the best move you can make to drastically lessen worry in your life. You may have heard this previously and never made a move on it yet trust me - it genuinely will spare you. Furthermore, on the off chance that you are not having a craving for dealing with yourself, ensure you are not building up an "I couldn't care less" frame of mind towards life that could cover an issue further than pressure.

## 5. Do less.

Truly. It's as basic as that. Do less and be increasingly lethargic. Train yourself to sit idle and be cool with it. One of the principle reasons why individuals load their day with errands to achieve, it's not on the grounds that they'll kick the bucket on the off chance that they don't complete them, this is on the grounds that doing heaps of things, going around, making telephone calls and noting huge amounts of messages make you feel significant. It makes you have an inclination that you are having any kind of effect, similar to you are in charge.

The best way to have a genuine effect is to make the most of each activity, be completely present and aware of the outcomes of every one of your activities. Concentrate on one errand at once, figure out how to organize and simply take the path of least resistance.

# CHAPTER SEVEN

## DEALING WITH STRESS

**1. Maintain a strategic distance from Caffeine, Alcohol, and Nicotine.**

Maintain a strategic distance from, or if nothing else decrease, your utilization of nicotine and any beverages containing caffeine and liquor. Caffeine and nicotine are stimulants thus will expand your degree of stress as opposed to diminish it.

Liquor is a depressant when taken in enormous amounts, however goes about as a stimulant in littler amounts. In this manner utilizing liquor as an approach to ease pressure isn't decisively useful.

Swap energized and mixed beverages for water, home grown teas, or weakened regular natural products squeezes and intend to keep yourself hydrated as this will empower your body to adapt better to pressure.

You ought to likewise plan to keep away from or lessen your admission of refined sugars - they are contained in many fabricated sustenances (even in exquisite nourishments, for example, plate of mixed greens dressings and bread) and can cause vitality crashes which may lead you to feel worn out and peevish.

When all is said in done, attempt to eat a sound, well-adjusted and nutritious eating routine.

## 2. Enjoy Physical Activity

Upsetting circumstances increment the degree of stress hormones, for example, adrenaline and cortisol in your body.

These are the "battle or flight" hormones that development has hard-wired into our cerebrums and which are intended to shield us from quick real hurt when we are under risk. Be that as it may, worry in the cutting edge age is infrequently cured by a battle or flight reaction, thus physical exercise can be utilized as a surrogate to use the unreasonable pressure hormones and reestablish your body and psyche to a quieter, progressively loosened up state.

When you feel pushed and tense, take an energetic stroll in natural air. Attempt to fuse some physical movement into your every day schedule all the time, either previously or after work, or at noon. Customary physical action will likewise improve the nature of your rest.

## 3. Get More Sleep

An absence of rest is a critical reason for pressure. Sadly however, stress likewise interferes with our rest as musings continue spinning through our heads, preventing us from loosening up enough to nod off.

Instead of depending taking drugs, your point ought to be to amplify your unwinding before resting. Ensure that your room is a quiet desert spring without any tokens of the things that reason you stress. Dodge caffeine during the night, just as extreme liquor on the off chance that you realize that this prompts aggravated rest. Quit doing any rationally requesting work a few hours before hitting the sack with the goal that you give your mind time to quiet down. Take a stab at washing up or perusing a quieting, undemanding book for a couple of minutes to loosen up your body, tire your eyes and help you disregard the things that stress you.

You ought to likewise mean to hit the hay at generally a similar time every day with the goal that your psyche and body become acclimated to an anticipated sleep time schedule.

## 4. Attempt Relaxation Techniques

Every day, attempt to unwind with a pressure decrease procedure. There are many attempted and tried approaches to lessen pressure so attempt a couple and see what works best for you.

For instance, attempt self-entrancing which is simple and should be possible anyplace, even at your work area or in the vehicle. One basic procedure is to concentrate on a word or expression that has a positive importance to you. Words, for example, "quiet" "love" and "harmony" function admirably, or you could think about a self-asserting mantra, for example, "I merit quiet in my life" or "Award me quietness". Concentrate on your picked word or expression; in the event that you discover your brain has meandered or you turned out to be mindful of nosy contemplations entering your psyche, essentially dismiss them and return your concentration to the picked word or expression. On the off chance that you end up getting to be tense again later, basically quietly rehash your statement or expression.

Try not to stress in the event that you think that it's hard to unwind from the start. Unwinding is an aptitude that should be learned and will improve with training.

## CONCLUSION

In conclusion dealing with stress can be a major challenge or tasks but gradually over a period of time you can learn how to cope with stress and strive to live a stress free. Always remember to take it easy on yourself and always strive to put a smile on your face.